NAVIGATING SWOLLEN LYMPH NODES WITH CONFIDENCE AND CARE

Discovering Resilience And Empowering Strategies For Confronting Challenges And Mastering Wellness

DR. WESLEY IAN

© [2024] [Wesley Ian].

DISCLAIMER

The information in this book is not meant to replace professional medical advice, diagnosis, or treatment; rather, it is meant mainly for general informational reasons. If you have any questions about a medical problem, you should always consult your doctor or another trained health expert. Don't ever discount expert medical advice or put off getting it because of something you've read in this book.

Any negative effects or repercussions arising from the usage of the material provided herein are not the responsibility of the book's author or publisher. It should be noted by readers that the material in this book is not all-inclusive and might not address every facet of the subject. Furthermore, new research may have an impact on how health concerns are understood or treated because medical knowledge is always changing.

No particular test, treatment, method, or product mentioned in this book is endorsed or promoted by the author or publisher. The reader assumes all risk associated with using the information included in this book.

Before making any big decisions regarding your health, it's crucial to speak with a licensed healthcare provider. The relationship between a patient and their healthcare practitioner should not be replaced by this book, nor is it meant to offer medical advice.

The opinions presented in this book are the author's and may not necessarily represent those of the publisher. Any errors, omissions, or inaccuracies in the information in this book are not the responsibility of the author or publisher.

It is recommended that readers independently confirm any information contained in this book and speak with a healthcare provider about their specific medical needs and state of health.

TABLE OF CONTENTS

ABOUT THE BOOK

The thorough manual Navigating Swollen Lymph Nodes with Confidence and Care is intended for anyone struggling to understand the intricacies of lymphatic system problems. This book is an invaluable resource for patients and medical professionals who want to learn more about enlarged lymph nodes and related disorders. It is based on a thorough investigation of the lymphatic system.

The book's goal is outlined in the preface, which also provides readers with a clear path forward. It explores the complexities of the lymphatic system, laying the groundwork for the chapters to follow. The fundamentals of lymph nodes, including their locations and activities inside the body, are explained. This foundational understanding prepares readers for a thorough examination of the causes of enlarged lymph nodes.

The reader is guided through the identification of enlarged lymph nodes by going over the symptoms, indications, and appropriate degree of concern. The book provides a comprehensive view by looking at common causes, enabling readers to make well-informed judgments regarding obtaining medical assessment and diagnosis, as explained in the following sections.

The book makes a distinction between benign causes and malignant disorders, such as autoimmune diseases linked to enlarged lymph nodes and cancer. The book offers insights into various treatment alternatives and approaches, which include drugs, surgical treatments, and complementary therapies. In addition, it highlights lifestyle management and self-care, including aspects of stress management, keeping a healthy lifestyle and monitoring changes.

The book also discusses support and emotional well-being, is a special feature of this book. It recognizes the psychological effects of lymphatic problems and offers readers' advice on coping mechanisms and creating a network of support. The significance of prevention and proactive health is emphasized. Readers are encouraged to adopt preventive measures, maintain a strong immune system, and schedule routine checkups.

Navigating Swollen Lymph Nodes with Confidence and Care is more than just an educational manual. It remains an indispensable ally, providing not only an abundance of information but also useful perspectives and consolation. For anyone looking for clarity and confidence in handling lymphatic system difficulties, this book is an invaluable resource.

CHAPTER ONE

INTRODUCTION TO SWOLLEN LYMPH NODES

KNOWLEDGE OF THE LYMPHATIC SYSTEM

An essential part of the human body, the lymphatic system helps with waste elimination, immunological response, and fluid homeostasis. Comprehending the lymphatic system is imperative to grasp the complex system of vessels, nodes, and organs that collaborate to promote general health and welfare.

AN INTRODUCTION TO LYMPH NODES

The lymphatic system is fundamentally a sophisticated network of blood-like tubes that run throughout the body. Lymph, a transparent fluid containing proteins, white blood cells, and other materials, is transported by these arteries. The lymphatic system, in contrast to the circulatory system, is propelled through its channels by muscular contractions and body motions rather than by a pump like the heart.

DESCRIBE LYMPH NODES

A vital part of the lymphatic system is the lymph nodes, which are tiny, bean-shaped structures placed thoughtfully all over the body. At lymph nodes, immunological responses are triggered and lymph is cleaned up, acting as vital filtering stations.

These nodes are essential to the body's defensive systems because they help recognize and fight poisons, infections, and aberrant cell growth.

THE BODY'S LYMPH NODES' FUNCTION

Lymph nodes are tiny, usually measuring between a few millimeters and a centimeter. They are dispersed throughout the lymphatic channels, gathering in particular areas to form clusters. These clusters are placed in key locations, including the neck, groin, armpits, and abdomen.

The way lymph nodes are distributed is indicative of how they monitor and filter lymph from various bodily locations.

Filtering and purifying lymph before it is reintroduced into the bloodstream is the main job of lymph nodes. Pathogens, other foreign materials, and cell detritus are carried by lymph as they pass through the lymphatic channels. As checkpoints, lymph nodes are places where specialized immune cells examine and react to the lymph's contents.

To neutralize a threat, immune cells within the nodes produce antibodies and trigger other defense processes in reaction to the detection of harmful chemicals.

WHERE THE LYMPH NODES ARE

Lymph nodes are arranged deliberately to cover different bodily parts. The cervical region of the neck has lymph nodes; the axillary region of the armpits contains nodes, and the inguinal region of the groin contains nodes. To ensure complete coverage, there are lymph nodes strewn across the thoracic and abdominal regions.

Comprehending the lymphatic system, the fundamentals of lymph nodes, their structure, and their role is crucial to understanding the complex processes that support the immune system and the general health of the body. An essential first line of defense, the dispersed network of lymph nodes aids in the body's capacity to recognize and fight infections.

CHAPTER TWO

IDENTIFYING INFLAMED LYMPH NODES

SYMPTOMS AND INDICATIONS

Lymphadenopathy, or swollen lymph nodes, is a common sign of an underlying medical condition. For prompt intervention and suitable medical care, it is essential to recognize the symptoms and indicators. The obvious swelling of one or more lymph nodes, typically found in the neck, armpit, or groin areas, is one of the main signs of swollen lymph nodes. Tenderness may accompany the swelling, which is frequently palpable.

Depending on the underlying reason, swelling lymph nodes can present with a variety of signs and symptoms. Localized pain or discomfort, redness of the skin above, and elevated body temperature in the affected area are examples of general symptoms. Additionally, the skin above the enlarged nodes may seem taut and glossy. People may have less range of motion in adjacent joints, and occasionally, additional symptoms like fever, exhaustion, or unexplained weight loss may coexist with the edema.

WHEN TO SHOW CONCERN

Accurately assessing when to seek medical assistance for enlarged lymph nodes is critical. While slight swelling may be a typical reaction to an infection, recurring enlargement or the occurrence of concerning symptoms call for additional research. Seeking medical attention is advised if the swelling is accompanied by excruciating pain, keeps getting worse over time, or is connected to symptoms that are not understood, including persistent fever or night sweats.

TYPICAL REASONS FOR INFLAMED LYMPH NODES

Lymph nodes that swell might occur for several frequent reasons. Bacterial, viral, and fungal infections can all cause lymphadenopathy, making infections a common cause. Swollen nodes in the neck or armpit areas can be caused by respiratory illnesses, including strep throat or colds, as well as skin diseases, like cellulitis. Enlargement of the lymph nodes can also result from sexually transmitted diseases like HIV or syphilis.

Lymph node enlargement can also be caused by autoimmune illnesses. Causes of lymphadenopathy include lupus, rheumatoid arthritis, and some forms of inflammatory bowel disease, which cause the immune system to react improperly against the body's tissues. Furthermore, as cancer cells spread throughout the lymphatic system, malignancies such as lymphomas and metastatic tumors may cause the swelling of neighboring lymph nodes.

Swollen lymph nodes are an uncommon side effect of some treatments, including some antiseizure meds and vaccinations. It may not always be possible to determine the source of lymph node enlargement, which calls for additional diagnostic research.

Identifying enlarged lymph nodes requires being aware of symptoms and indicators that can point to an underlying medical condition. It's important to know when to seek the right medical assistance, especially if symptoms increase over time or persist. Many infections, autoimmune diseases, and cancers are among the major causes of enlarged lymph nodes, which highlight the significance of a comprehensive medical evaluation to determine the underlying cause and carry out a successful treatment plan.

CHAPTER THREE

MEDICAL ASSESSMENT AND PROGNOSIS

SEEING A MEDICAL EXPERT

Most commonly, the process of seeking medical examination and diagnosis starts with a visit to a healthcare provider. This first phase is very important since it entails a thorough evaluation of the patient's past medical history, present symptoms, and pertinent personal data. To ascertain the nature of the illness and any potential risk factors, the healthcare provider converses with the patient during the consultation to obtain relevant information.

DIAGNOSTIC PROCEDURES AND TESTS

To accurately diagnose patients and identify underlying health conditions, diagnostic tests, and procedures are essential to the medical evaluation process. Common diagnostic procedures like blood testing might reveal important details about a patient's health. These tests can determine the quantity of particular compounds, count blood cells, and find out if there are any antibodies or infectious agents present. Healthcare practitioners can learn a great deal about a patient's general health and spot any anomalies by examining the blood's composition.

IMAGING RESEARCH

Imaging investigations are a vital part of medical diagnosis in addition to blood tests. To view internal structures and spot anomalies, these examinations make use of cutting-edge technology like computed tomography (CT) scans, ultrasound, magnetic resonance imaging (MRI), and X-rays. When assessing the health of soft tissues, bones, and organs, imaging examinations are especially useful since they help medical practitioners identify cancers, fractures, and other structural abnormalities.

AUTOPSY

Another diagnostic technique used to gain a deeper comprehension of aberrant tissues or lesions is a biopsy. A biopsy involves taking a small sample of tissue for microscopic analysis from the afflicted area. Infections, autoimmune diseases, and malignancies are frequently diagnosed using this process. Different forms of biopsies, such as needle biopsies or surgical biopsies, may be performed depending on the nature of the suspected illness.

A comprehensive consultation with a healthcare professional is the first step in the complicated process of medical examination and diagnosis. Blood tests, imaging investigations, and biopsies are examples of diagnostic tests and procedures that are essential in determining the complexity of a patient's health. These resources support healthcare providers in creating treatment plans that are suited for each patient's unique needs in addition to helping to identify current health conditions.

CHAPTER FOUR

CAUSES OF SWOLLEN LYMPH NODES THAT ARE NOT SERIOUS

INFECTIONS

Numerous non-serious reasons might result in lymphadenopathy or swollen lymph nodes. A typical reason is infections, which fall into two categories: viral and bacterial. When dangerous germs are present in the body, the immune system reacts by inflating the lymph nodes, which can result in bacterial infections. This reaction can be brought on by illnesses like strep throat, bacterial skin infections, or tooth infections, which expand and tenderize the lymph nodes. The enlarged lymph nodes themselves are frequently a transient and benign sign of the body's attempts to fight the infection, even if these illnesses may need medical intervention.

BACTERIAL DISEASES

Likewise, viral infections can result in the swelling of lymph nodes. Viruses, such as the flu, mononucleosis, and the common cold, boost the immune system and cause lymph nodes to expand. Swollen nodes might be the result of lymphatic system inflammation brought on by the body's immunological reaction to viral invaders. After the viral infection is treated, the lymph nodes usually shrink back to their original size. While swollen lymph nodes are frequently caused by infections, it's vital to remember that not all diseases create this symptom, and the severity might vary.

HYPERSENSITIVITY

Another non-serious reason for enlarged lymph nodes is allergies. Allergens like pollen, pet dander, or specific foods can cause the immune system to react, which can lead to an inflammatory response that enlarges lymph nodes.

The body is trying to get rid of or neutralize the perceived threat by triggering this reaction. In general, allergic reactions are not dangerous on their own, and lymph nodes frequently shrink back to their usual size if the allergen is eliminated or treated.

CONDITIONS INFLAMMATORY

Infections or allergies unrelated to inflammation can also cause enlarged lymph nodes. The immune system misattacks healthy tissues in autoimmune diseases like lupus and rheumatoid arthritis. Lymph nodes may be affected by this ongoing inflammation, which could result in swelling. The enlarged lymph nodes are frequently a subsequent reaction to the underlying inflammatory illness, even though these conditions may need constant care.

A wide range of benign reasons, including bacterial and viral infections, allergies, and inflammatory diseases, can induce swollen lymph nodes. It is essential to recognize the many causes of lymphadenopathy to distinguish between benign and potentially dangerous underlying conditions. Although enlarged lymph nodes are often a transient and reactive reaction, cases that are persistent or severe should be assessed by a medical practitioner to rule out any potentially dangerous underlying disorders.

CHAPTER FIVE

SEVERE ILLNESSES AND DISORDERS

THE LYMPH NODES AND CANCER

Understanding the link between cancer and lymph nodes is essential to comprehending how cancers spread and advance inside the human body. As a component of the lymphatic system, lymph nodes are essential for capturing and filtering dangerous materials, such as cancer cells. Lymphatic veins can be invaded by cancer cells, which cause neighboring lymph nodes to expand. Swollen lymph nodes are frequently a sign that cancer may be present in the body, requiring more testing and diagnosis.

CANCER TYPES LINKED TO INFLAMED LYMPH NODES

Swollen lymph nodes are a prominent indicator of cancer's involvement in the lymphatic system and are frequently linked to different forms of the disease. Cancers that commonly cause swelling of the lymph nodes include melanoma, lung cancer, breast cancer, and lymphoma, a kind of blood cancer that starts in the lymphatic system. The identification of enlarged lymph nodes frequently aids medical practitioners in determining the fundamental cause of the cancer and formulating a suitable course of treatment.

SETTING AND HANDLING

A crucial part of diagnosing and treating cancer is staging, which sheds light on the scope and gravity of the illness. It entails figuring out the tumor's dimensions, whether it has affected neighboring tissues, and whether it has progressed to distant organs or lymph nodes. Treatment selections are frequently impacted by the stage of the disease, which is determined by the presence of cancer in lymph nodes. Cancer patients may receive chemotherapy, radiation therapy, immunotherapy, surgery, or a mix of these treatments. The objective is to stop the cancer from spreading, eradicate it, or manage it, and enhance patient outcomes overall.

IMMUNE SYSTEM DISORDERS

The term "autoimmune diseases" refers to a group of illnesses in which the body's immune system unintentionally targets healthy tissues and cells. Damage to many organs and systems as well as persistent inflammation might result from this abnormal immune response. Many different types of autoimmune disorders can impact almost every area of the body, including the internal organs (such as lupus), joints (such as rheumatoid arthritis), and skin (such as psoriasis).

DIABETIC ARTHRITIS:

The joints are the main organs affected by rheumatoid arthritis (RA), a systemic autoimmune disease. The synovium, the membrane lining surrounding joints, is the target of the immune system, which results in inflammation and damage to the joints. Symptoms of RA include stiffness, deformity, edema, and discomfort in the joints. Effective disease management requires early diagnosis and response. Rheumatoid arthritis treatment strategies include taking antirheumatic drugs (DMARDs) to reduce inflammation, changing one's lifestyle to improve general health, and taking medications to relieve symptoms.

LUPUS

Systemic lupus erythematosus (SLE), sometimes known as lupus, is a complicated autoimmune disease that can impact several organs and systems, such as the kidneys, skin, joints, and heart. Antibodies produced by the immune system target healthy tissues, causing inflammation and damage.

Numerous symptoms, including fever, rashes on the skin, exhaustion, and joint discomfort, are indicative of lupus. Medication for lupus treatment usually consists of immunosuppressants, anti-inflammatory medicines, and lifestyle changes to control symptoms. A multidisciplinary approach and consistent monitoring are crucial for managing the many lupus symptoms and enhancing the quality of life for those who are impacted.

OPTIONS AND STRATEGIES FOR TREATMENT: ANTIBIOTICS

Medications are essential for treating a wide range of illnesses because they provide a variety of choices for symptom management and healing. One family of drugs called antibiotics is mostly used to treat bacterial infections. They function by either eradicating bacteria or preventing their proliferation. Antibiotics are frequently given to treat ailments like skin infections, lung infections, and urinary tract infections. They are essential in the removal of bacterial pathogens from the body. However excessive use of antibiotics can result in antibiotic resistance, which highlights the significance of prudent prescription and treatment regimen adherence.

ANTI-INFLAMMATORY MEDICATION

Another class of pharmaceuticals is anti-inflammatory ones, which work to lessen inflammation and its accompanying symptoms. NSAIDs, or nonsteroidal anti-inflammatory medications, are commonly used to treat fever, inflammation, and discomfort. They work by preventing the synthesis of prostaglandins, which are important inflammatory mediators. NSAIDs are frequently used for ailments like rheumatoid arthritis, musculoskeletal traumas, and other inflammatory diseases. When using these medications over a lengthy period, it is important to take into account potential adverse effects, especially those that may affect the cardiovascular and gastrointestinal systems.

PROCEDURES SURGICAL

A vital component of medical care is surgery, which is frequently required when more conservative methods are insufficient to manage a patient's condition. Minor operations like excisions and biopsies to big interventions like organ transplants or joint replacements can all be considered surgeries. Surgical techniques seek to remove sick tissue, fix anatomical anomalies, or return the body to its natural functioning. Modern surgical methods, such as minimally invasive treatments, have reduced recovery periods and minimized postoperative problems while also improving patient outcomes.

ALTERNATIVE AND COMPLEMENTARY MEDICINE

Complementary and alternative therapies are a broad category of unconventional methods intended to improve general health and reduce symptoms. Acupuncture, chiropractic adjustments, herbal remedies, and mind-body practices like yoga and meditation are some examples of these therapies. Many people use complementary and alternative therapies to treat various ailments, even though some of them lack strong scientific backing. Integrative medicine has grown in popularity as a holistic approach to patient treatment that addresses the mental, emotional, and spiritual dimensions of health by combining conventional and complementary therapies.

There is a wide range of therapeutic choices and techniques available, with drugs serving as a fundamental component for the management of a variety of medical disorders. Certain components of infectious and inflammatory processes are the focus of antibiotics and anti-inflammatory medications, respectively. When it comes to treating serious illnesses and anatomical defects that call for immediate action, surgical procedures are essential. In addition to conventional treatments, complementary and alternative therapies provide individuals seeking holistic approaches to health with more options. Optimizing treatment outcomes requires a thorough and customized approach that takes into account the unique requirements and preferences of each patient.

CHAPTER SIX

EMOTIONAL HEALTH AND ASSISTANCE

HANDLING THE EMOTIONAL IMPACT

People's ability to deal with life's experiences and obstacles is influenced by their emotional health, which is a critical component of general health. Managing the emotional effects of different circumstances is essential to preserving mental health.

This process entails identifying and comprehending one's feelings, permitting appropriate expression, and figuring out practical stress-reduction strategies. Coping strategies can take many different forms; they can include anything from relaxing and joyful activities to mindfulness and meditation.

Coping methods include critical elements such as self-awareness and resilience building, which enable people to face and constructively regulate their emotions.

PUTTING TOGETHER A SUPPORT NETWORK

It is impossible to exaggerate the significance of having a strong support network for emotional health. Human ties are essential for offering consolation, empathy, and support when things are hard.

Cultivating meaningful relationships with friends, family, and other people who can provide empathy and support is a crucial part of creating a support system. T

hese relationships provide a safety net, enabling people to live in a setting where they are respected and understood. Good communication is essential in a support system because it enables people to share their experiences, express their emotions, and get validation. Maintaining these relationships promotes a sense of community and belonging in addition to improving mental health.

SEEKING PROFESSIONAL ASSISTANCE

Although personal networks offer beneficial support, there are times when obtaining professional assistance is required to preserve emotional health. Psychologists, counselors, and therapists are examples of mental health specialists who have the training and experience to help people with more difficult emotional problems. Knowing when to get professional assistance is a sign of strength since it shows that one is committed to maintaining their mental health.

Depending on the type and intensity of emotional problems, professional help may involve counseling, therapy, or psychiatric treatment.

Through the therapy connection, people can explore their feelings, gain understanding, and create coping mechanisms that are specific to their situation in a private, judgment-free environment.

Developing emotional well-being requires a multimodal strategy that includes managing the emotional effects, creating a strong support network, and, if needed, obtaining professional assistance.

People can develop resilience, improve relationships with others, and more easily manage the complexity of their emotions by incorporating these ideas into their daily lives. Setting emotional well-being as a top priority promotes not only personal fulfillment but also the development of a compassionate and understanding community that cherishes its members' mental health.

CHAPTER SEVEN

PROACTIVE HEALTH AND PREVENTION

SUSTAINING IMMUNE SYSTEM HEALTH

A strong immune system is essential for general health and is vital in preventing a wide range of illnesses and infections. Proactive health requires adopting a lifestyle that strengthens and supports the immune system. Sufficient sleep, a balanced diet, and regular exercise are all crucial for keeping the immune system strong. Frequent exercise increases immune cell circulation and strengthens the body's defenses against infections. The vitamins, minerals, and antioxidants found in a well-balanced diet provide the body with the fuel it needs to perform at its best.

Furthermore, a strong immune system is a result of practicing mindfulness and relaxation practices to manage stress.

FREQUENT MEDICAL EXAMINATIONS

Proactive steps are taken in preventive healthcare to detect and treat possible health problems before they worsen. The foundation of preventive care is routine health examinations, which enable people to track their health and identify any early warning indicators of disease. These check-ups frequently consist of physical exams, tests, and consultations with medical specialists. Regular health evaluations can help detect diseases like diabetes, hypertension, and some types of cancer early on, allowing for prompt treatment and control. Beyond targeted screenings, routine examinations promote a proactive attitude toward health by motivating people to be in constant contact with their healthcare providers and take an active role in their health.

IMMUNIZATIONS AND PREVENTATIVE STEPS

Immunizations protect a range of infectious diseases, making them an essential part of preventative healthcare. Vaccines prime the body to fight against particular diseases by inducing an immunological response from the immune system without actually producing the sickness. Immunization reduces the spread of infectious illnesses by protecting individuals as well as enhancing community immunity. Comprehensive preventive care requires following advised immunization schedules, such as those for hepatitis, measles, and influenza. Apart from immunizations, the body's defenses are further strengthened and health risks are reduced by implementing preventative actions including maintaining proper hygiene, abstaining from tobacco and excessive alcohol use, and employing protective measures against environmental threats.

Promoting resilient and thriving well-being requires giving priority to preventative and proactive health measures. A complete approach to wellness involves accepting immunizations and preventive measures, scheduling routine health check-ups, and fostering a healthy immune system through lifestyle choices.